BARIATRIC SURGERY

The Complete Gastric Sleeve Guide

David Harris

© Copyright 2016 By David Harris

© Copyright 2016 by David Harris - All rights reserved.

This document is geared towards providing exact and reliable information in regards to the topic and issue covered. The publication is sold with the idea that the publisher is not required to render accounting, officially permitted, or otherwise, qualified services. If advice is necessary, legal or professional, a practiced individual in the profession should be ordered.

From a Declaration of Principles which was accepted and approved equally by a Committee of the American Bar Association and a Committee of Publishers and Associations.

In no way is it legal to reproduce, duplicate, or transmit any part of this document in either electronic means or in printed format. Recording of this publication is strictly prohibited and any storage of this document is not allowed unless with written permission from the publisher. All rights reserved.

The information provided herein is stated to be truthful and consistent, in that any liability, in terms of inattention or otherwise, by any usage or abuse of any policies, processes, or directions contained within is the solitary and utter responsibility of the recipient reader. Under no circumstances will any legal responsibility or blame be held against the publisher for any reparation, damages, or monetary loss due to the information herein, either directly or indirectly.

Respective authors own all copyrights not held by the publisher.

The information herein is offered for informational purposes solely, and is universal as so. The presentation of the information is without contract or any type of guarantee assurance.

The trademarks that are used are without any consent, and the publication of the trademark is without permission or backing by the trademark owner. All trademarks and brands within this book are for clarifying purposes only and are the owned by the owners themselves, not affiliated with this document.

Introduction

I want to thank you and congratulate you for downloading Bariatric Surgery: The Complete Gastric Sleeve Guide.

This book serves as a guide for those considering bariatric sleeve surgery for themselves, or for those who have already been approved for the procedure. It is a collaboration between the author and a bariatric surgery patient's personal experience. Content will be delivered directly from the first-hand account of the patient where ever appropriate.

I underwent the procedure in 2013 and have assembled this book as a resource for those who are skeptical about the procedure, or are simply looking for information to make a more informed choice. Bariatric surgery is not for everyone, and even those who qualify for the procedure may find that there are better options that suit their needs. It is an extreme step taken for weight loss reduction, but for many the benefits to one's health and wellbeing far outweigh any potential negatives of the surgery.

The material in this book will fulfill all of your needs for not only researching gastric sleeve surgery, but will also feature my own personal experience with the process. My own story will be kept to a minimum, and I will mainly draw on my experiences to paint a clearer picture of what you can expect. It is important to note that this book is written from the perspective of the American healthcare system, and so some notes on costs, doctors, and locations for the procedure may differ from your own country. This procedure has become standardized over the last ten years and much of the information will still be useful if you are outside of the U.S., but purely from the perspective of healthcare costs, you will be gaining insight into the American healthcare system.

If you are not undertaking bariatric surgery, this book will serve the purpose of assisting in research and for aiding in the decision making process for a loved one considering the procedure. The benefits of bariatric surgery are immense. So many of the mid to late life health problems are based on medical complications from excess weight. From diabetes to heart disease, to greater instances of cancer, being overweight is simply not a healthy lifestyle. In addition to physical ailments, there is also the mental toll of being overweight. Depression and anxiety are highly correlated with obesity and often these ailments go untreated as patients seek to not treat these serious mental disorders.

It is my hope that by completion of this book you have all of your questions about gastric sleeve surgery answered. From the benefits and disadvantages of the procedure, to the costs and medical history of the surgery, you will have a clear picture of what to expect both before and after the procedure. It's time to make an informed decision, to know what the future holds for you or a loved as the choice is made whether to undergo surgery. Continue reading and have all of your questions answered, including ones that you may not have yet considered.

Table of Contents

Introduction i
Table of Contents v

Chapter 1: Background & History 1
Mechanism And Function Of Sleeve Gastrectomy 3

Chapter 2: The Qualifications for Surgery 7
Do You Or A Loved One Qualify? 7
A Note About The BMI 11
My Own Story 12

Chapter 3: Making An Informed Choice 17
Advantages 17
Disadvantages 21

Chapter 4: Preparing For Surgery 25
Diet Prior To Surgery 25
Insurance And Costs: 26
Meeting With Doctors 27
Surgery And Recovery Location 28

Chapter 5: Day Of The Surgery 29
From The Patient's Perspective 29
Discharged 32
General Expectations In The Week Post Surgery (Physician-dependent) 33
Reason For Concern 34

Chapter 6: Life Post-Bariatric Surgery 37
Pain 1 To 3 Months Post Surgery 37
Diet After 1 Month 38
Diet After 6 To 8 Months And Beyond 39
Weight Loss In The Long Term – Plateaus And Avoiding Old Habits 40

Conclusion 43

Chapter 1: Background & History

Current day bariatric surgery is the culmination of research and the development of procedures during the mid-twentieth century. During the 1950s, open procedures on the stomach were conducted for a variety of specific health concerns. These ranged from bile duct stones to blockage in the lower intestines. The reasons for surgery early on were not related to obesity or meant with the intent of having a patient lose weight. It was during these early days that the foundation of intestinal surgery was formed. Techniques for reaching the intestines and colon were developed to solve these specific health concerns, but in this research and development came anastomosis. This is the cornerstone of current day bariatric sleeve surgery and wouldn't be possible without the techniques developed during this time.

Anastomosis is the process of connecting two disparate sections of the body, after removing a section in between that was the source of an ailment. In the stomach and intestinal tract this was done for treating specific illnesses. Parts of the intestines or stomach needed to be removed as they were the sites of ailments. Using this technique, a surgeon could reconnect two parts of the stomach or intestine and they could serve the same function. At the time this was a medical breakthrough. The ability to have a functioning intestinal tract while still removing a large section of the stomach was a difficult process to master, and in addition to advances in surgical tools there was a steep learning curve for surgeons willing to undertake the procedure in these early days of surgical operation.

In recent decades the advances set about in the middle of the last century led to procedures specific to the function of losing weight. There is little doubt that you are familiar with the term 'stomach stapling', as this was the first common procedure practiced, and it gained prominence in the 1990s. This procedure is not all that different from current day bariatric band surgery, however several steps required for stomach stapling have been removed. In addition, the main implant to control the size and flow through the intestine has been adjusted to a duodenal switch. This relatively simple implant functions as an elastic band placed near the top of the intestine, after a large section has already been removed. It is a far cry from the early days of the procedure and works not only in the same mechanism as stomach stapling, but allows for a far less invasive surgery and has reduced costs significantly. Today, it is the most expensive of the three most common surgical options, with gastric sleeve surgery being the cheapest. The band can be loosened if needed, and it is placed in such a way that adjustments can be made easily and with a short minimally invasive process.

The surgery as we know it today, serves the primary function of aiding a patient to lose weight by shrinking the total size of the stomach by around seventy percent. There is a range in how much of a reduction is done to the stomach, in extreme cases the stomach being reduced by an overall of eighty five percent. Intuitively, you know that this means the patient cannot ingest as much food, but in addition to the pure physical reduction, there is a far more important change that takes place. It reduces the production of ghrelin, a hormone that stimulates hunger. This severe reduction leads a patient to not develop the cravings for food that led to their significant weight gain.

Mechanism And Function Of Sleeve Gastrectomy

Bariatric sleeve surgery is an offshoot of gastric bypass surgery and the later development of the adjustable gastric band. This surgery is the fastest growing stomach surgery in western countries, with a high success rate among patients losing weight and keeping it off for life, based on present day survey data. A large portion of the stomach is removed and the surgery is not reversible. This differs from use of the gastric band as a smaller section of the stomach would be removed, and over time the remaining section could inflate if a patient is not careful with their dietary habits. The more extreme measure in bariatric sleeve surgery results in greater instances of patients losing weight in the long term, however data sets, while robust, do not feature a number of years in the same way that earlier stomach procedures do.

The surgery is almost always conducted with a small incision in the abdomen. From here, laparoscopic tools are used to remove a section of the stomach through the small incision. This is a major factor for why the surgery has risen to prominence in recent years. Laparoscopic surgery uses tools with fiber optic cameras that are moved through the body through a small incision instead of requiring a large, open incision. The advantages here cannot be understated. It reduces the costs significantly, as well as the recovery time and instances of complications. Much of the problems stemming from open surgery are rarely the procedure itself, but rather the risk of issues stemming from the invasive incision in the abdomen. It requires a different degree of anesthesia and greater surgical mastery of the procedure. That is not to say that current day bariatric sleeve surgery is a simple process, but rather that it has come a long way from the early days of reducing a patient's weight through surgery.

The high success rate using a sleeve in bariatric surgery, along with the relatively low cost, has led to a large increase in the practice. This in turn has led to further reductions in cost as the procedure has become standardized. Very recently, in the last three years, the surgery has become popular in eastern countries as obesity cases are on the rise. The success rate of the surgery, measured in weight loss, is extremely high, with patients losing around fifteen pounds per month on average. This number varies greatly from patient to patient depending on their starting weight, gender, and height.

The wide spread practice of the surgery has seen a great increase in the number of patients that qualify. The

Body Mass Index (BMI) of a patient is typically over 40, however in recent years this has fallen to a range of 35-40, and there are some advocate groups that would like to see the surgery practiced on BMIs even lower than 35, depending on patient history. The age requirements for the surgery have also fallen in the last five to seven years, with the procedure now being recommended to patients as young as fourteen. However it is applied far more commonly to patients eighteen years and older. Certain groups have made a case for the procedure being done on patients younger than fourteen, however the pushback has been far greater than in the advocacy of surgery on those with a BMI of 35 or less. It is worth noting that most doctors do not recommend bariatric surgery lightly, and it is still seen as an extreme measure to combat complications from obesity. Comorbidities, that is two diseases present in a patient, raise the frequency of recommendation of bariatric surgery. It was not long ago that comorbidities would disqualify patients from bariatric surgery, however due to the non-invasive nature of bariatric sleeve surgery; it is highly recommended to patients suffering comorbidities.

Chapter 2:
The Qualifications for Surgery

Do You Or A Loved One Qualify?

It's a complicated question that needs to be discussed with your primary care physician; however there are some guidelines that could get the discussion started. Patients who qualify for bariatric sleeve surgery are typically eighteen or older, and have a BMI of 35 or above. Outside of the BMI scale, a patient that is over 400 pounds will almost certainly qualify, as this is the cutoff where the surgery is deemed to be at its safest. I was under this weight when I underwent the surgery, and it is quite possible a different doctor would not have recommended the procedure based on my weight. A patient should have tried numerous ways to lose weight in the past, typically by modifying their diet and including exercise in their weekly routine. Bariatric sleeve surgery recovery is a short period of time, and the costs are fairly low, but that does not mean it is not still a mentally and physically taxing procedure, as well as costing what amounts to a large sum of money for many families. It is always recommended that a patient attempt to diet and exercise before considering surgery, and that they understand surgery is simply an aid to losing weight and not an immediate solution that requires no effort on the part of the patient.

If a patient has tried diet and exercise but has struggled to lose weight, then bariatric surgery might be the answer. Once surgery is complete, then a patient must stick to a strict diet to get the proper nutrition. The extreme reduction in the size of the stomach will reduce weight, but the cost is that anything a patient eats becomes all the more important. A patient will still need a daily allowance of iron, vitamins, and other minerals, and getting all of this while reducing their caloric intake by some eighty percent is not an insignificant challenge. One must be prepared to follow a strict dietary regimen, and so undertaking the surgery does not mean a patient gets to eat what they please. In many ways this dietary restriction is significantly more difficult to maintain than to simply lose weight through regular diet and exercise.

The screening process for bariatric surgery can take up to half a year, and during this period a physician will monitor your progress in following dietary restrictions. Since following a strict regimen post-surgery is so important to getting the essential nutrients that one needs, a patient must demonstrate that they can follow such guidelines before the surgery. This means that a patient will likely lose weight prior to surgery by simply following the guidelines of their doctor. It is understood that a patient is inherently having trouble with their weight and that not all of these guidelines will be followed day in and day out, but certain changes in a patient's weight will almost certainly disqualify a patient from surgery. Weight gain during the screening process is one such disqualifier; this is a sign that a patient is unwilling to commit to certain dietary restrictions and is unfit for surgery. It may also signal to medical professionals that the patient does not have the right viewpoint on the surgery overall. The mental wellbeing of a patient is one of the qualifiers for surgery, and they must understand that bariatric surgery truly is a tool to weight loss, and little more. This is part of the reason why bariatric surgery for young adults and minors is somewhat controversial, as the idea that they can fully internalize the importance of the surgery is up for debate; they are young enough in their lives that they should pursue more traditional weight loss methods. For some, getting cleared for surgery can instill an idea that they suffer from a chronic disease of obesity, while this isn't far from the truth in pure physical symptoms and conditions, it sometimes has a patient label themselves as obese. A patient self-identifying as obese is an additional warning flag for medical professionals. It signals that surgery is not a solution to the core problem of a patient and that therapy and other forms of behavioral treatment may be better suited for aiding a patient.

If you or a loved one suffer from physical ailments due to being overweight then this increases the chances of qualifying for surgery. Early symptoms of diabetes are very reversible (as is late stage diabetes but to a lesser degree), and bariatric surgery increases the chances of maintaining good health and reversing these symptoms. More complicated and nuanced ailments like early signs of heart disease, high blood pressure, and weak joints and bones are also signs that a patient may qualify for surgery, however these are altogether harder to qualify. They are merely indicators of greater health risks down the line, such as increased risk of heart attack and stroke. For a young patient, such as a teenager, they may not have many of these symptoms or health conditions, but there is still reason for looking into surgery to reverse the mental toll of being overweight.

Obesity is highly correlated with anxiety and depression. In the formative years of a teenager, such mental ailments can become lifelong conditions that lead to difficulty in every aspect of daily life, ranging from employment opportunities, to forming friendships and more. This is an extremely nuanced issue, and if you are a parent considering the options of surgery for your son or daughter, you will want to confer with them to check the status of their mental health. Relay this information to their primary care physician to better determine if bariatric surgery is right for your family. While the expenses and recovery from the surgery can seem extreme, in comparison to the lifelong issues stemming from mental health conditions, it may be in the best interest of your family to commit to surgery. These are all things to take into account as you determine whether or not to pursue this avenue of medical treatment. It is an extremely difficult decision to undergo surgery if a patient is under the age of eighteen, and even at this early stage of adulthood it can be difficult to find medical professionals willing to commit to the surgery. This is changing, but the increased prevalence of doctors willing to suggest surgery for minors and young adults will only continue to increase over time. It is because of this changing viewpoint that you may want to seek medical professionals specifically tuned to treating minors, knowing that a decade from now it is likely that your current doctors would be more willing to recommend the procedure, and that you are merely thinking down the line.

Even for non-minors, most doctors will not recommend surgery for patients until they have tried diet and exercise for a number of months, and even then there is a prevailing attitude in the medical community that unless medical issues stemming from obesity are life threatening, they should not undergo surgery. If you truly believe that surgery is the best chance to successfully lose weight, then consider visiting another doctor. This may seem like going around your primary care physician, and indeed it is, but when the prevailing attitude does not allow for surgery, you may have to take action into your own hands and find a doctor willing to aid you and your family in this venture. I mention this from my own personal experience, as it was a multi-year long process until my doctor acquiesced and was in favor of bariatric surgery. If this would be the end result all along, then it would have been beneficial to undergo the surgery earlier. It would have been better for my health overall and I sometimes think about the time that I missed out on by desperately trying to lose weight through traditional means.

A Note About The BMI

The BMI scale is an inherently flawed way to measure obesity, however it requires just two measurements and is the most common form of measurement. The BMI does not take into account muscle mass or bone density. If you are obese on the BMI scale, but used to lift weights, you will find that the BMI may not accurately reflect the degree in which you are overweight. This is a key aspect of determining if a patient qualifies for surgery, so make sure that you speak with your medical professional and determine the degree to which you or a loved one are overweight. More importantly, post-surgery and as a patient measures their success in weight loss, strength training will become an important component in maintaining good health. Here is where the BMI scale can sometimes scare patients into thinking that they are at more risk than they truly are – a patient should keep this in mind as they gain muscle mass, since the BMI scale will become more and more incomplete in describing a patient's overall weight as it relates to their height. Progress made post operation should be measured by how a patient feels, their energy levels, and how their prior existing conditions are regressing. They should not just rely on the BMI scale to determine the overall success of their weight loss endeavor.

My Own Story

I do not wish to dwell on my own life for too long, but I did want to include a very short synopsis of my medical history and how I came to undergo bariatric sleeve surgery. I insert this story as an anecdote for how someone can determine that the surgery might be right for them, as well as the costs and the recovery process. It was a complex decision that involved my doctor and my family, as well as a long period of introspection. There was a period before undergoing surgery that I thought I was giving up, or giving in to being obese. It led to mental health issues as well as the early symptoms of diabetes. Let this serve as a guide for how someone can determine for themselves if bariatric surgery is right for them; it is not going to be a one story fits all guide, but does give some idea for how one can go down the road to surgery.

I started to develop issues with my weight when I was in middle school, around the age of thirteen to fourteen years old. I was overweight during this time, but not classified as obese. It wasn't until around the age of twenty that I started to be classified as obese. During college my BMI was hovering around 37 to 38. I was obese by any standards, but I was surrounded by friends and familiar faces; the weight truly did not bother me and did not impede my ability to live a productive life.

Post graduating college my weight went up to 342 pounds – the heaviest I ever was in my life. I'm five foot, seven inches, and this extreme weight led to issues in my everyday life. I was twenty-five years old and working my first job for a large company. Getting up every morning was a struggle as my weight made me more tried than I would have been. It was around this time that I started to discuss surgery with my doctor. I had heard about gastric surgery using a band – there was a television special that covered it on 60 Minutes. It would be an additional year until my doctor told me that I would qualify for this surgery, but recommended gastric sleeve surgery instead. The primary difference being in the success rate, where patients who went with the later surgery typically kept the weight off for the duration of their lives. Band surgery has higher instances of patients gaining some weight back, as the band can loosen and the stomach can expand unless the patient adheres very strictly to a new diet.

I was screened for the surgery and put under a new diet by my doctor. This diet was a macro breakdown of carbs, protein, and fat. It was in a specific ratio to help me adjust to what would be my new diet post operation. It took roughly three months for my insurance to clear paying for the operation in any capacity, although the out of pocket costs would top eight thousand dollars when all was said and done. The surgery was a relatively painless process, and I was discharged from the hospital two days after the operation.

Over the next two years I lost 140 pounds. My symptoms of diabetes reversed within the first eight months and the only long term negative effects came in the form of excess skin all over my body. This is one of the major consequences of all forms of gastric bypass surgery, and is merely a fact of losing weight. The more quickly that weight is lost, the greater the excess skin sags on the body. In my own circumstance, this has started to improve in the last year. Strength training is a major contributor to reducing the excess skin on the body, and today I feel comfortable with my appearance both in the workplace and out.

There are a few notes that I want you to take away from this story. First, while most patients that undergo surgery weigh in excess of 400 pounds, depending on height of the patient as well as the attitude of the doctor, patients that weight less may still qualify, as was my case. Second, although it led to me losing a tremendous amount of weight, it is not as though the process was immediate. It would be nearly a year until I felt noticeably different, even though I was losing lots of weight every single month. The final takeway is that issues regarding weight stem from the mind, and I needed to be in good mental health to undergo the procedure. I had to have the right attitude about what my life would be like afterwards, and that it wasn't a cure all for many of issues of the mind that led to my weight gain to begin with.

Chapter 3: Making An Informed Choice

Bariatric sleeve surgery is not a perfect solution to obesity, but truly no options are perfect. There are many advantages specific to surgery and it is important that you and your family are fully aware of what is at stake. Life post-surgery is an adjustment to normal activity, and making an informed choice requires all of the facts and information. As you read this chapter and look through the advantages and disadvantages, I can't stress enough that my overall view is that bariatric sleeve surgery pros outweigh and potential disadvantages. From experience, one must go into this endeavor with the right viewpoint, and the only way to solidify that picture in an accurate way is to have as much information as possible.

Advantages

Effectiveness:

Patients typically lose sixty percent of their excess body weight in the first two years post-surgery. This is with following strict adherence to the dietary regime prescribed by medical professionals.

Qualifications:

Many patients will qualify for this type of surgery, and even if one doctor does not clear a patient, a different doctor is likely to approve of bariatric surgery. This is not going around a doctor so much as it is finding one that is more up to date with the current medical practice of bariatric surgery. In addition, the age of a patient can be as young as fourteen, although it is typically not done on patients younger than eighteen to twenty years old.

Reverses Conditions Related To Obesity:

Comorbid conditions related to obesity are typically reversed within the first year following surgery. This is variable depending on the conditions and the age of the patient, but overall the point is that severe issues stemming from obesity are reversible and do typically start to reverse in the first year. The advantages of this are plain to see, but they also include added benefits like not needing to take diabetes medication, as well as reduction in needing to take medication for high blood pressure.

Success Rate:

The success rate of patients that have undergone bariatric sleeve surgery nears one hundred percent. A patient will lose weight in the year to two years post-surgery and the rate of weight loss is at about 15 pounds per month, although this number is highly variable depending on the starting point of the patient. Where the success rate is not so clear is in the long term outcomes of patients. The data here is just not available for the long tails on how patients do with diseases relating to obesity. While the current view is that most diseases are reversible with the surgery, there is a real possibility that the stomach will expand over time. This expansion will overall be far less than if the patient had undergone bariatric band surgery, and the stomach will never reach the original size prior to operation, but one must be aware that success rates in the long run (20-30 years) are currently unknown.

Reduced Instances Of Obesity Related Medical Conditions

Bone and Joint Issues: Long term obesity damages bones, causing micro fractures and reducing bone strength overall. In minor cases this simply causes discomfort, but in greater cases it increases the risk of greater injuries to bones and joints.

Hypertension: Associated with many long term health conditions, ranging from heart attack to stroke, hypertension is a clear sign of poor health. High blood pressure forces the heart to work harder, and while the exact causation for how hypertension relates to most heart related illnesses is still debated, the correlation is clear – hypertension results in long term health consequences that are debilitating to living a normal life, and can be life threatening.

Sleep Apnea: Obesity is associated with higher instances of sleep apnea; that is the body not getting enough oxygen during sleep. At the very least, patients with sleep apnea report being more tired during the day because the quality of their sleep at night is poor. In worse circumstances, it increases rates of heart disease and stroke. In the worst case scenario, sleep apnea can cause sudden death during sleep, however this last case is rare.

Diabetes: 29 million people in the United States have diabetes – it is one of the most common chronic diseases today. The long term health consequences of type two diabetes are higher rates of heart attack and stroke. Patients must monitor their blood sugar levels several times per day and may become reliant on insulin to control their blood sugar. In rare cases it can lead to blindness or loss of a limb.

Mental Health Issues: The mechanism is not at all clear for many of the mental health issues associated with obesity, however among obese populations there is a greater rate of depression, anxiety, bipolar disorder, and schizophrenia. Often these issues go untreated for years, or are never treated at all. In addition, there is some level of eating disorder associated with many that suffer from obesity.

Recovery Time:

The recovery time of the surgery is just one to two days in the hospital post-surgery. Following this period, the patient must follow a strict diet to ensure that they are getting the proper nutrition based on their limited caloric intake. They are able to return to work one to three weeks post-surgery, depending on their field. The patient cannot participate in heavy lifting (greater than 10 pounds) for six weeks post operation. All of these are extremely minor inconveniences for this type of surgery. Most importantly, a patient undergoes this surgery without a large incision. Instead, a small incision can be made in the abdomen and tools with fiber optic cameras can complete the surgery in around two hours.

Cost:

The overall cost of this surgery is relatively low, with an average out of pocket cost of $14,000. This is a large sum of money, but in comparison to the cost of health complications from obesity it is extremely minor. In addition, insurance companies are increasingly covering part of the cost of this procedure. From the viewpoint of an insurance company, covering the cost of surgery now means reduced costs in the long run care for that patient.

Disadvantages

Cost:

It cannot be ignored that the cost of surgery is rarely fully covered through insurance. While the cost in the long run is far less than treating all of the complications that form from obesity, the price of surgery is still far greater than losing weight through diet and exercise. Diet and exercise will always be the preferred method of weight loss whenever possible.

Strict Dietary Restriction:

Post-surgery, a patient's diet will consist of liquids for two weeks. They will then move on to a soft mush style of food, similar in texture and form to baby food. A patient will then move onto soft foods and eventually around the one month mark be able to eat solid foods. The major disadvantage here is that the reduction in the size of stomach means that everything a patient eats becomes far more important. They will need to get the right amount of nutrition from the food that they do consume, and cannot rely on eating more of one particular food to get vitamins and minerals. The diet will be far stricter than trying to lose weight in a natural way.

In addition, eating in general is very difficult for a patient. It can be painful to eat a meal as the stomach recovers from surgery. Patients often have to force themselves to eat to ensure that they are getting the right nutrients.

Sagging/Excess Skin:

The major disadvantage of bariatric sleeve surgery is the excess skin that will sag when a patient loses weight. The degree to which this both bothers patients, and in how much skin sags, is highly variable on the individual. The degree to which the skin sags is both a function of the patient's age and height, as well as external factors like how their skin has been stretched over the years. Most patients will suffer from some degree of excess skin as weight is lost. It causes some degree of discomfort for patients, but mostly it is the mental picture that patients have of themselves that suffers most. Patients must be aware that this is one of the steps in the recovery from bariatric surgery, and cannot be avoided. Additionally, sagging skin would develop if a patient lost weight by more traditional methods.

There are a couple of different ways in which a patient can combat excess or sagging skin. For one, several months after surgery they should start weight training. This will expand the muscles and tighten the skin in the process. Two, a separate purely cosmetic surgery is available if the patient wishes to go this route. This surgery is fairly expensive, is not covered by insurance, and offers no health benefits aside from the mental wellbeing of the patient.

Potential Complications From Surgery:
Complications from bariatric sleeve surgery are exceedingly rare, but when they do occur they are very serious. There are three primary complications that one must worry about. All of these complications have severe consequences if not treated immediately, however they are very rare because of the non-invasive nature of the surgery. The complications are internal bleeding, abdominal infection, and complications from the anesthetic used during surgery.

Internal bleeding is the most common of these complications, but again it happens very rarely. This occurs when there is a leak from the staple near the cut of the stomach. This leads to internal bleeding from the stomach to the mid-section of the body. This complication is why patients need one to three weeks for post operation recovery depending on their field of work, and also why they cannot lift objects heavier than ten pounds for up to a month. As long as a patient avoids breaking these suggestions as set forth by their doctor, then internal bleeding should not occur. If it does happen, a patient must go to the hospital immediately. They will become aware of this complication by experiencing strong pain in their abdomen.

Abdominal infection could stem from the surgery itself, but is rare because of the small incision that is cut in the abdomen. This complication stems from poor disinfection protocols of the tools used during the operation, and would be the fault of the medical team conducting the operation. Major precautions are taken in hospitals so that this does not happen, and instances of this are very rare. This can be treated with antibiotics but will require a patient to visit a hospital to find why the problem occurred. A patient would become aware of this complication very shortly after surgery, as they would develop a fever, as well as severe pain in the abdomen.

The most severe complication of this surgery is related to the anesthesia used. A patient is fully under anesthetic during the operation, and if the wrong amount of anesthetic is used then the patient can fall into a coma. This is a worry of all operations that require a patient to be fully asleep during surgery, and instances of this are exceedingly rare in every country, but especially in the United States and European countries. It is something a patient should be made aware of, but nothing that should cause them to not to go through with surgery.

Chapter 4:
Preparing For Surgery

Diet Prior To Surgery

Preparing for surgery is a multistep process that is both physically and mentally demanding. Once a patient has been approved for surgery by their doctor, they will be given a strict diet regimen to follow. A patient must follow this diet precisely as veering from it could disqualify them from the procedure altogether; this is done to ensure that a patient can follow even stricter dietary restrictions post operation. A patient will meet with his or her doctor with greater frequency, checking their vitals and ensuring that they remain in good health to undergo the surgery.

During this time, it is quite possible that depending on how a patient's weight is fluctuating with the dietary restrictions, doctors will recommend that a patient does not undergo surgery. This is actually quite common, and if a patient is losing weight steadily through diet, then the surgery is avoided altogether. In most circumstances, a patient loses some weight and they still undergo the surgery. In the immediate weeks leading up to surgery, a patient will need to follow a specific set of dietary restrictions. These are extreme and the patient will have every meal outlined for them. This is to ensure that the patient can undergo the surgery with little issue or complications, and is a necessary step in going forward with the procedure. The diet will consist primarily of lean proteins with a severe reduction in carbohydrates. There is an emphasis on a severe reduction in sugar, as in none that is added to any food eaten by the patient. Depending on the surgeon, the 48 hours leading up to surgery may have further dietary restrictions. Almost always this consists of a total elimination in solid foods. A patient will subsist on water, Jell-O and depending on the surgeon's instructions, one protein shake per day. The patient is also to eliminate caffeine and carbonated beverages two days prior to surgery.

Insurance And Costs:

The out of pocket costs for bariatric sleeve surgery are around $14,000, although this number is variable depending on the quality of insurance of a patient. In my own case, my insurance company covered enough of the cost to bring down my out of pocket costs to $8,000. This covers some, but not all, of the treatment required. Post operation a patient will require a very special blend of nutrients; this is actually a prescription medicine but is relatively affordable, although again it varies depending on insurance.

It is quite possible that a patient's insurance company will refuse to pay for bariatric surgery upon first request. In this case an appeal can and should be made. An American patient with any degree of insurance should have some of the cost reduced. A patient typically needs to make a case to the insurance company for why they should pay for it, and the argument typically is that paying for surgery would reduce the long term healthcare costs for a patient. Sometimes this argument is made through an employer if that is the source of healthcare coverage for a patient.

Some patients may find that traveling to another country can reduce the cost of surgery significantly, similarly to getting plastic surgery in a foreign country. While bariatric sleeve surgery has become common practice in western countries and in parts of Asia, it is still far from a standard procedure in many places. It is highly suggested that a patient not go this route, as the maintenance required following surgery is extensive, with checkups and dietary advice needed from medical professionals.

Meeting With Doctors

A patient will meet with their team of doctors prior to surgery. This includes the full team that will aid the patient during their surgery, from the anesthesiologist to the surgeon. This is done primary for the benefit of the patient and to build trust between the patient and the team of doctors. The meetings between the whole medical team before surgery is very brief, and can be as close to surgery as the morning of the operation. Various appointments are made ahead of time to check the weight of a patient, and to read vitals over a series of several weeks, but this is usually done by nurses. On the morning of surgery, or sometimes the night before, a patient will meet their operating room nurse. This nurse will be with them all through recovery in the hospital, as well as prepping them for surgery before they go under.

Surgery And Recovery Location

The surgery in America is done exclusively in hospitals. While the surgery has become quite standardized, it is still a major surgery that requires an anesthesiologist and a set of specialized medical equipment nearby in case there are complications. The hospital where the surgery is performed is typically the one closest to the patient, however this may differ depending on insurance. Some new policies will incentivize patients to have the surgery done at a hospital where the prices are more favorable for the insurance company. In some cases, a patient may have to travel some distance to a hospital where the surgery is done, or to where a team has more experience with the surgery. For many surgeons, this is a procedure that is routine, and one that they have conducted in the past.

Recovery for the surgery is typically one to two days in the hospital where the surgery is done. This depends on a few different factors, such as the age and gender of the patient. Typically, women will have a slightly longer recovery time. It is not a function of the insurance of a patient, however a patient may need to increase their out of pocket expenses to extend their stay at the hospital.

Chapter 5:
Day Of The Surgery

From The Patient's Perspective

For most that undergo the bariatric sleeve surgery, they will arrive at the hospital the morning of their surgery, just a few hours before the surgery is to take place. Depending on the insurance policy and the hospital, a patient may spend the night prior to surgery at the hospital. This is largely done to make sure that the food they ingest is safe for the anesthetic the following morning. For the most part though, this is very rare. The surgery is almost always done in the morning, sometime before noon.

You feel nervous and perhaps a bit anxious, but you should not worry. This is a very routine surgery and the complications that could appear won't happen during the surgery itself. If there are any issues at all, it will happen a few days after the surgery is complete, and it can't be stressed enough, these complications are incredibly rare. As you come into the hospital, it is important that you have followed your surgeon's diet precisely, and that you have not added any medications or drugs that were not previously approved by medical staff. If for some reason you took a medication that was not approved by your doctor, including minor drugs like aspirin, you must tell the hospital staff before entering the operating room. The major one that people forget about is tobacco, for wish of not having their insurance company find out. A patient must make sure to specify if they have used tobacco in any regard prior to entering surgery.

Once you go to hospital admitting, they will direct you to the pre operating section. Here you will meet the nurse that will be with you in the operating room. She will be your guide for the next two days, the one that walks you through both the process leading up to surgery as well as the recovery in the hospital after the operation. You will discard all of your clothing, watches, and jewelry and change into your hospital gown. You will have already met your surgeon and anesthesiologist in most cases, but if you have not they will introduce themselves at this time. Even if you met him or her in the past, your anesthesiologist will make another appearance prior to you going under. Your operating nurse will give you something to calm you down, as well as hook you up to an IV. The wait time in the pre operating room is kept to a minimum, as your surgery will have a definite scheduled timetable to follow.

As you make your way to the operating room proper, expect to be wheel chaired around. This is done in many hospitals in the United States for insurance reasons; patients that slip and fall may sue the hospital and administrators want to avoid this. In the operating room itself, you should be feeling nice and calm from what your nurse gave you. You will then have a facemask put on and told to count back from ten. And that's it; that is all you need to do prior to surgery. At this time the surgeon will be operating on you, and this will take around one to two hours.

When you wake up, you will be in the recovery ward of the hospital. It's likely that you see your surgeon again that day, letting you know how your surgery went. Your operating nurse will assist you with most everything that you need. You will be allowed to see your family, but expect to be very drowsy and just generally fatigued. You should only have minor pain in your abdomen, if any at all. Usually during the visiting time, or a little while after, your operating nurse will have you walk around for just a few minutes. This is to get your blood flowing and avoid clots. The end of your first day will come shortly after, as you'll be so tired from the drugs and surgery.

How long you stay in the hospital is dependent on a few different factors, but primarily it is your age and gender. Women tend to need more time in the hospital, as well as older individuals. The stay at the hospital post-surgery is done to make sure that there are no complications, and if there are then these will crop up within just a couple of days of surgery. Your insurance policy also plays a little bit of a factor here, but the hospital will not discharge you until it is safe for you to return home. If your stay at the hospital is only approved for one day post-surgery according to insurance and you need an additional day in the hospital, expect additional expenses to come out of pocket. That, or you may end up fighting it out with your insurance company after the fact. The cost per day in the hospital is extremely expensive, ranging anywhere from five thousand to ten thousand per day, and even then the cost is really hard to determine. Rates at the hospital are so highly variable and even within the same hospital in the same room; the cost could vary purely based on what billing department chooses to charge you. We shouldn't stress this point too much, but most expenses come from the seemingly random costs charged by the hospital billing department. Don't worry too much about this aspect, and know that if you do get charged anything out of pocket, nothing is actually set in stone. These prices are highly negotiable.

Discharged

Returning home from the hospital, you will need to rest for, at minimum, a full week. You will be given some pain medication to treat any abdominal discomfort that you feel, but expect this to actually be quite minor; you think it will feel worse than it actually does. You will be on a strict diet, following guidelines of no carbonated beverages and no caffeine. You cannot eat solid food and instead will be subsisting off of liquids for the following week. In the immediate few days after you get home, it will be more Jell-O and water, as well as a mix of vitamin pills prescribed by your doctor. I was given a prescription shake to take for a full week after my surgery. Simply follow your doctor's orders and make sure not to eat any solid or semi-solid foods. The passage leading to your stomach is significantly constricted, as well as sore. Swallowing solid food might not make its way past this constricted section of your stomach, making it extremely painful and will result in another trip to the hospital.

General Expectations In The Week Post Surgery (Physician-dependent)

Liquids:

Sip liquids frequently for a full week after surgery. Your nurse in the hospital will remind you to do this, but you will need to stick to it after you get home as well. It may feel as though you are quite full from just a little bit of water, but keep on drinking. You are going to be very dehydrated from surgery and need as much liquid as possible. Sip small amounts throughout the day to make this process easier.

Bowl Movements:

Bowl movements will be painful for up to a full week after the surgery. This is completely normal part of the process and is no reason to worry. In addition, depending on the type and amount of painkillers prescribed, it may be difficult to pass a stool at all.

Stomach Pain:

Expect stomach pain that feels like mild heartburn after you get home. It's no reason for concern and is going to develop from a buildup of stomach acid. Depending on the severity of the pain, you may need Protonix to reduce the acid buildup. If the pain increases, call your doctor and see if this medication is right for you.

Movement:

Do not be sedentary during your recovery period. Even during that first week home you will want to move around quite a bit. Take it easy and commit to walks of ten to fifteen minutes at a time. This will speed up the recovery process significantly. Expect there to be some pain in the first couple of days that you are moving around.

Fatigue:

You can expect to be quite exhausted during your recovery, and this could be for up to a full month post your operation. This makes sense; your calorie intake has been slashed significantly. You simply aren't giving your body the same amount of energy through food as you used to. This a normal part of the process and your energy levels will come back with time, although typically on the order of a few months.

Cleanliness:

You will not be able to take a bath for about three weeks following surgery. You can shower but the tub is going to be out of the question.

Contact Your Surgeon If You Need To:

Do not hesitate to contact your surgeon if you have any sort of emergency or have any questions. Some feel timid about contacting their surgeon, but this is their job and they fully expect post op patients to check in. This is especially true if you have any of the following symptoms in the next section.

Reason For Concern

Instances of complications from bariatric sleeve surgery are very rare, but they can occur. You will want to contact your surgeon immediately if you suffer from any of the following:

- Pain that increases with intensity over a period of 24 hours.

- Nausea that is constant, and starts one to two days after you've returned home.
- If you are unable to swallow liquids. This one is very serious and should only develop in the immediate hours following your surgery. This is typically tied to inflammation in the esophagus or near where the sleeve is placed on your stomach.
- A high fever with chills and shaking, similar to a bad case of the flu. This is a sign of infection and even if unrelated to the operation, must be discussed with your surgeon.
- A buildup of pus around the sites of the incision on your abdomen. Even without pus, contact your surgeon if you feel warmth near the incision sites lasting more than two hours, accompanied with redness of the skin.

Chapter 6:
Life Post-Bariatric Surgery

Pain 1 To 3 Months Post Surgery

A patient can expect minor pain and swelling for up to three months post-surgery. The pain should be minor, but still noticeable, especially when partaking in any sort of physical activity that stretches or contorts the abdomen. This will subside as the weeks go on, and by around the three month point a patient will no longer need pain medication.

In today's climate with the increased awareness of the dangers of pain medication, it is doubtful that a doctor would issue a prescription for very long. A patient should follow their doctor's recommendation about what pain medication to take and with what frequency. They shouldn't try and tough it out, but it's important to note that taking medication for a long period of time can cause minor symptoms of withdrawal once the medication is fully removed from a patient's regimen.

An additional note is that for the first week or two that a patient significantly reduces their pain medication;

they can expect rapid changes in their bowl movements. A patient will be on medication for a minimum of three weeks and this long period of time creates a constant state of constipation for the patient. This will subside but it does so in a fairly rapid way; it's something that should be expected but not something that is all too disruptive to a patient's life.

Diet After 1 Month

At around the one month point, a patient will start to consume solid foods again. They must not be overly acidic, and they must be taken with a fair amount of vitamin pills. These are special supplements that are prescribed by a patient's doctor, and are a necessity to ensure the proper nutrition for a patient. A patient must also continue to drink lots of water; much of the water that was obtained by the patient before the surgery was received through the solid food they were eating. While solid foods are back in the diet, they are consuming far fewer calories and need to supplement this with an increase in liquids.

It is possible that even when a patient is ready to consume solid foods, it will be difficult. This comes from the shrunken stomach, but also from the pain and swelling of the passage leading to the stomach. If solid foods are difficult to eat, a patient should blend them with fat free milk, water, or broth. For many, broth preserves some of the flavor that is otherwise lost when blending with other liquids And if hot broth is used, it helps to soften the foods even more. It is not suggested that a patient uses a straw to consume these liquids as often the suction causes pain in the esophagus; a result of the swelling from the surgery of the stomach and a slight buildup of acids around the lower section of the throat. For most, at around the two month point this additional restriction of no straws can be removed.

Energy levels during this period are still diminished from a lack of calories being taken in, however patients typically experience extra energy from the quick rate of weight loss in these early months. The body is starting to get into a state of ketosis; that is burning fat instead of glucose for energy. This is variable depending on the age of the patient, the physical activity they get post-surgery, as well as the state of their liver. Healthier livers are more efficient at having the body gain energy from ketosis.

Diet After 6 To 8 Months And Beyond

At around six months, a patient will switch to their maintenance diet. This is the beginning of the learning process for how they will eat for the rest of their lives. In addition to the doctors a patient is already familiar with, a nutritionist is also involved. At this stage, it is the nutritionist who actually becomes one of the most important medical professionals for a patient. They will calculate the macros that a patient needs, as well as assist in determining the vitamins and supplements that are needed. Beyond eight months, appointments with a nutritionist will be consistent, but not as frequent as once a month. The macros for a diet typically do not change that much after the eight to nine month range, and instead it is about ensuring that a patient can maintain their current diet and have enough energy throughout the day. Modifications are made based on the amount of physical activity and energy levels of the patient.

A patient will feel very full from what are very small amounts of food. This is because of the shrunken stomach, but also because some degree of swelling still exists. This is a great time to develop new habits, typically behavior that is the opposite of what caused a patient to need bariatric surgery in the first place. Eating slowly and savoring every bite is a key component of these new eating habits. Typically, a patient would have eaten much faster leading up to surgery, rarely savoring the taste of food and instead going for volume. Trying to keep this habit going post-surgery is a recipe for extreme stomach pain as more food can be ingested before it is sensed by the body that it simply cannot contain that much volume.

This is a great time to also start learning how to cook and become more intimate with food. Part of the issue with eating disorders is that abstinence is not a solution like for other behavioral addictions. A healthy relationship must be maintained with food as it is something that cannot be cut out completely. In addition, when and with whom a patient eats is a factor in their success. Eating should be an activity to itself, and should not be done on the run or in front of a computer or television. Good eating habits start with eating at the same time each day and using it as a time for the family to discuss their day.

Weight Loss In The Long Term – Plateaus And Avoiding Old Habits

The weight loss that a patient experiences is a reason for joy, but after the two year point there will be a plateau. This is not inherently a bad thing, and the patient is still going to be losing weight, albeit at a far slower rate. The issue is it can be difficult for a patient to adapt to the mental challenges of this slower rate of change. Bariatric surgery is a tool to assist in weight loss, but is a not a solution by itself. A patient must be willing to make long term changes in their relationship with food and how they incorporate exercise into their life. It will be impossible for a patient to go back to their old weight, but it is quite possible to have a patient revert to their old mindset. Sticking to a diet, changing one's relationship with food, and adding exercise to their routine is the only surefire way to avoid old habits that led to bariatric surgery and the poor mental state associated with it.

Conclusion

It's my hope that the information in this book helps you in making an informed decision about bariatric sleeve surgery. If you or a loved one suffers from obesity, there are many different options available for treatment. Surgery should be thought of as a last resort, but it can be a useful tool in extreme cases of morbid obesity. In situations where comorbidities exist in a patient, surgery can often slow, or altogether reverse the progression of these diseases.

Obesity is a lifelong disease. It can be treated with surgery, but that does not treat the very heart of the disease. If you or a loved one decides to have bariatric sleeve surgery, it will not solve each and every problem. The physical aspect of obesity cannot be ignored, and for this, bariatric surgery is an indispensable tool with an amazing success rate and very few instances of complications. It will aid in all physical aspects of the disease, but patients will still need to work through the longer term issues that caused their obesity. They will need to adhere to a strict diet and incorporate exercise into their lives.

You should now have enough information to make an informed choice for you or a loved one. Be sure to weigh the pros and cons of the surgery, and know that as someone who has undergone the surgery himself, it is not going to be for everyone. It should only be used in the most extreme of cases, and for those who have already tried other ways to lose weight. I have no doubt that I would be in far worse health had I not received the surgery some three years ago. From the possible complications associated with the surgery, from taking time off work, to medications, to the monetary cost of the surgery itself, I do not regret my decision. This is a difficult choice to make, but you now have the knowledge to make the right choice.

CPSIA information can be obtained
at www.ICGtesting.com
Printed in the USA
LVOW10s2000200417
531570LV00016B/833/P